Potato Diet for Beginners:

Comprehensive Guide on Potato Diet or Meals; What to Eat & What Not To Eat, Pros & Cons, Health Benefits of the Regimen, Different Recipes, FAQs & Answers and Lots More

By

Élodie D. Archambault

Copyright@2024

TABLE OF CONTENTS

CHAPTER 1

INTRODUCTION

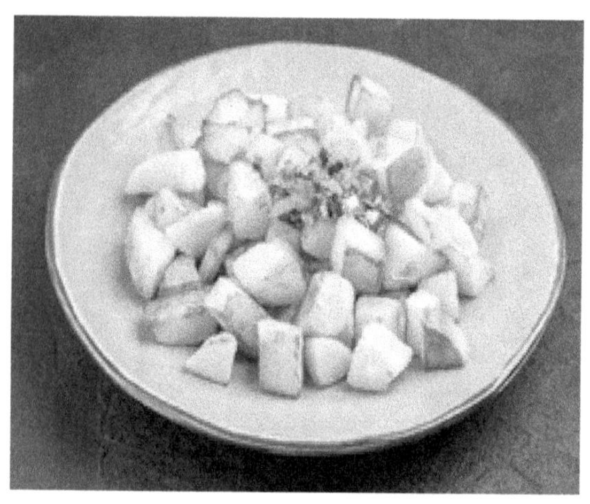

What's the potato diet?

The potato diet serves as a fast weight loss plan. This diet relies on potatoes for calories. The potato diet assists to help you lose a pound weekly by providing fiber, vitamins, and minerals.

Many forms of the potato regimen involve eating only potatoes for a period of time. Due to its restrictions, this diet should not be followed long-term.

What Studies Say

Like a cabbage soup nutrition, grapefruit diet, and others, the potato diet prioritizes weight over health. The restricted diet can lead to disordered eating by not satisfying nutrient demands, instilling dread of specific foods, cutting out huge groupings of foods, including eating from a list of 'allowed' foods rather than following your body's cues.

Amazingly, if you want to achieve a weight loss within a short-term, then this is your sure bet!

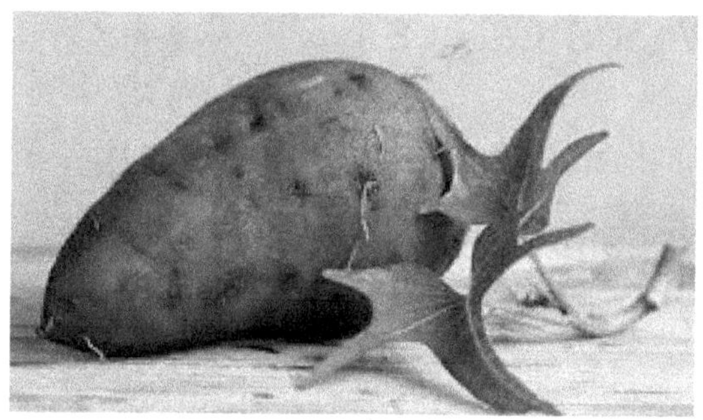

CHAPTER 2

POTATO DIET: FOODS TO EAT AND THE ONES TO AVOID RIGHT AWAY

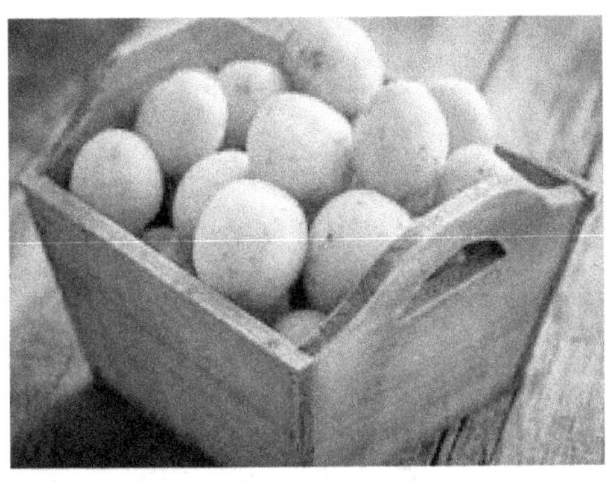

What One Can Eat

Potato diets vary, but they all are vegan, minimal in fat, and promote eating till full rather than weighing quantities or counting calories.

Potato diets promote bulk eating. Fill up on low-calorie meals from nature. While eating less calories during the day, consuming a lot makes you feel full.

Plain Potatoes

Different potato diets allow different potato varieties. Some demand white potatoes alone. A more permissive variant allows yellow, red, as well as sweet potatoes.

Whole, Low-Calorie Plant-Based Foods

The pure potato diet forbids any other foods, even nutrient-dense fruits and vegetables.

Long-term sustainability is the goal of looser potato diets. Unprocessed foods may be allowed on the potato diet, depending on the version.

Potatoes should dominate your plate even when other foods made from plants are allowed. Potatoes should be supplemented with these nutritious meals.

Produce: Fruit, Vegetables, Legumes, Grains.

Spices and condiments

The stringent potato diet limits condiments, sauces, and seasonings. Small amounts of low-fat mustard plus homemade ketchup are permitted in less rigorous versions.

Salt can be used to season potatoes, although it's not

recommended. Condiments as well as seasonings should be fat-free and limited.

Drinks

Only water, simple coffee, and simple tea are permitted on the potato regimen. On and off a potato diet, drink lots of water to stay hydrated.

What Not to Eat

Some foods are allowed on the Potato Diet, depending on the variation. The harshest potato diet involves eating just potatoes for days.

Added Fats

Fats like vegetable oils are banned on the potato diet, like animal products. The potato diet emphasizes low-fat, thus extra fats are prohibited. Even modest amounts of extra fats pile up quickly because fats are high in calories.

Healthy fats aid potato nutrition uptake. Since it's meant to maximize weight loss quickly, the diet prohibits additional fats like:

Butter, vegetable oil, nuts, seeds

Processed as well as refined foods

The potato diet recommends eating complete, unadulterated foods. This excludes processed foods, which may be heavy in calories, fat, as well as sodium. They have fewer nutrients than entire foods. Despite being potato-based, baked potatoes are healthier than French fries, chips, and tater tots.

Pasta Bread Chips

Muffins

Doughnuts

Cereal Crackers

Animal Products

Potato diets are vegan in all forms.
All animal-based foods are
banned on the diet.

CHAPTER 3

MERITS AND DE-MERITS OF POTATO DIET PLUS PREARATION TIPS

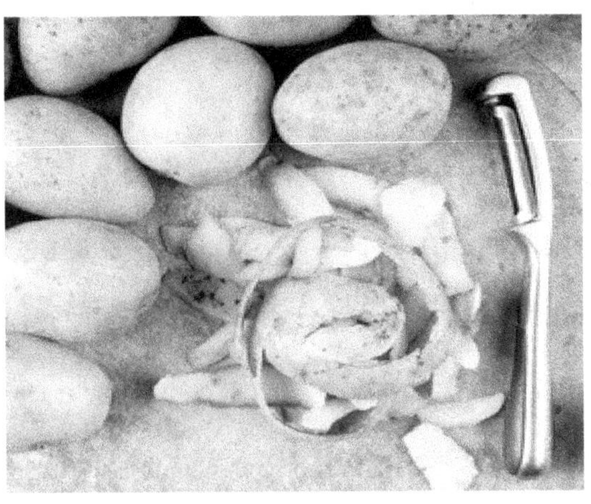

Potato Diet Pros

Potatoes lower fat and sodium and may help you lose weight

temporarily. However, this diet has minimal health benefits. Potatoes are healthful, but they should be part of a balanced diet with vegetables, fruits, whole grains, proteins, as well as healthy fats.

Possible loss of weight: The potato regimen is designed to lose weight. Natural low fat and calorie content makes it effective. Since the diet is strictly adhered to for a few days, loss of weight may not be sustained.

Short-term: The potato diet lasts two to five days, which may suit fast-trackers. Some advocates claim you can drop 1 pound every day, but this is unrealistic.

Some choose the potato regimen for weight loss and digestion. Potatoes are easy to digest, making this diet mild on the gut. Potatoes are high in fiber, which aids digestion.

Easy to adhere to: Mono diets including the potato diet are the easiest to follow. What is allowed and prohibited on the diet is clear. Simple diets like the potato diet are good for people who struggle with sophisticated ones.

Potato Diet Drawbacks

Potato diets pose health hazards and other downsides like previous fads.

One-food diets, especially root vegetables, are unsustainable. The potato regimen is an immediate trend, but some devotees have eaten just potatoes for a year. This diet is unsustainable for most people.

Diet lacking balance or variety: On the potato diet, many nutritious foods are banned. While potatoes are nutritious, they lack some

critical elements. The potato diet
might cause nutritional deficits
over time.

Expect short-term weight loss:
Short-term fad diets might not
maintain weight loss. This might
indicate water weight, not fat loss.
Returning to your usual lifestyle
may cause you to gain or regain
the weight that you lost on the
potato diet.

Potatoes are not nutritionally
balanced, thus they hinder healthy
eating. Nutrient-dense diets
include several foods, while potato
diets allow solely potatoes. Only

consuming one food may cause disordered eating.

Potato Diet Preparation and Tips

No meal schedule is defined for the potato diet. Breakfast, lunch, supper, and snacks are allowed because followers can eat till they're full. Short-term weight loss is the goal of the potato diet. This diet is usually followed for between two and five days, but others follow it for a week.

The type and preparation of potatoes are equally significant. Frying is discouraged. Use fat-free cooking methods include boiling, steaming, baking, as well as roasting.

Individuals determine what amount of potatoes to eat daily. Since most potato diets encourage eating till full, the amount varies for each person. Two to five pounds of potatoes daily is recommended. This diet is restricted, thus adherents may not acquire adequate nutrients should they consume too few calories.

Add veggies, fruits, grains, and legumes to the potato diet for balance and sustainability. Naturally low in fat, these foods are high in protein, vitamins, minerals, and fiber.

Dietary fat is essential to a balanced diet, but a quick-fix potato diet discourages it. Zero-fat diets are unsustainable.1 Add nutritious oils including nuts, seeds, along with avocado to a potato diet-inspired meal.

Since potatoes are cheap, the potato regimen is economical.

Conventionally farmed potatoes are cheaper than organic. This diet does not necessitate eating organic potatoes, but those who wish to limit pesticide exposure can.

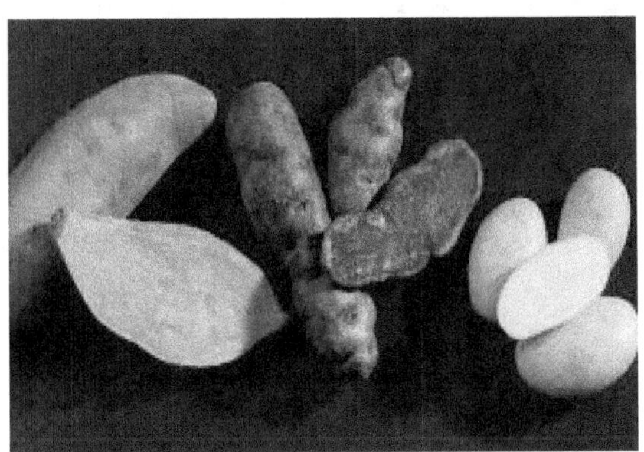

CHAPTER 4

POTATO DIET RECIPES YOU WILL REALLY LOVE

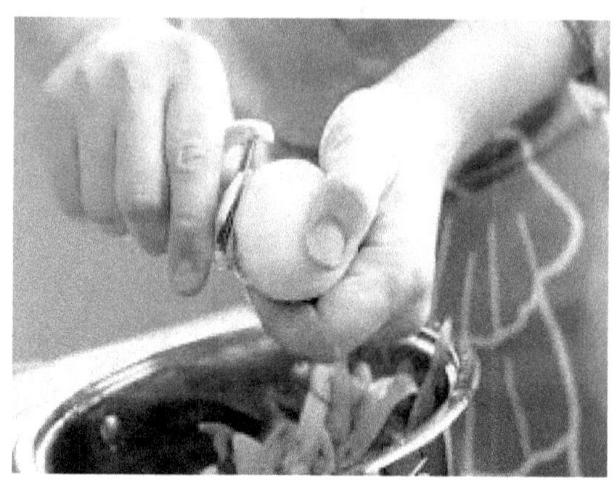

Healthy Potato Recipes

These fast, easy, and tasty healthy versions of fries and potato skins are healthful.

Root veggies stand out for their starch

Potatoes are veggies, but they're primarily carbs, thus they're not on any "healthiest foods" lists. The USDA reports 164 calories plus 37 milligrams (g) of carbohydrates in a medium russet potato containing the skin. The same-size portion of spuds contains 5 g of protein, 4 g of fiber, no harmful fats, plus a variety of B vitamins along with potassium.

While all white-fleshed potatoes are nutritionally similar, they have diverse tastes and textures that suit different meals. Russet potatoes are ideal for baking because of their very light, fluffy flesh. Yukon gold potatoes are inherently buttery and great for creamy mashed potatoes. Baby or miniature potatoes may be ideal for your meal if size matters. Whatever type you offer, potatoes in their natural state are healthful.

How potatoes are served is the issue. These tubers are mostly eaten as chips made from potatoes, French fries, or just other processed foods in the US. A USDA report found that 69% of potatoes sold were processed between 2020 and 2021. Prepared foods often add salt and fat and remove fiber.

Potatoes remain longer than most vegetables and neutralize many flavors. They're cheap, filling, and varied enough for daily eating. Remember to portion them like spaghetti, not lettuce. These dishes will teach you how to eat healthier potatoes.

These nutritious and fast recipes are explained below:

i Roasted potatoes, onions, and carrot

Simple Herb-Roasted Potatoes as well as Vegetables

Nothing is simpler or tastier than roasted veggies. This tasty side dish is enhanced by carrots, zucchini, plus onion to balance the potatoes' starchiness. Even on a busy weekday, this vegetable meal pulls together fast using pantry seasonings.

Ingredients

1 pound baby potatoes

-Slice a medium-sized red onion into wedges and cut 4 medium carrots into sticks with skin on.

-1 medium zucchini, cut rounds

-2 tablespoons extra-virgin olive oil

-3/4 tsp kosher salt

-Half a teaspoon of newly ground black pepper

-Optional fresh parsley garnish

Directions:

a. Pre-heat oven to 400°F.

b. Wash and fork-prick potatoes well. Place on a plate that is microwave-safe and microwave at high power for 3 minutes.

c. Add vegetables on top of a parchment-lined baking surface with potatoes. Toss using olive oil, pepper plus salt.

d. Bake 30–35 minutes until vegetables are tender and golden.

Nutritional Info

Per-serving calorie count

Total fat: 125

5g saturated fat

0.7g protein

Contains 2g of carbs.

20g fiber

3.2g sugar

3g added sugar

Zero grams of sodium, 196mg.

ii. Baked Garlic-Parm Fries

French fries are deep-fried, adding
calories and fat to a fat-free dish.
This dish uses extra-virgin olive oil
and an oven instead of a fryer.
Research suggests leaving the

potato peel on because it includes half the fiber. According a recent study, fiber aids regularity, decreases cholesterol, and regulates weight and blood sugar. Parmesan cheese brings rich flavor without many calories.

Ingredients

-4 medium russets

-2 tablespoons extra-virgin olive oil

-One teaspoon of garlic powder

-Kosher salt

-Finely ground black pepper

-3 tablespoons grated Parmesan

-2 tablespoons fresh parsley,
optional garnish

Directions:

a. Preheat oven to 425°F.

b. After washing the potatoes, cut
them into ½"-wide strips, leaving
the skin intact.

c. Pour olive oil over fries in a big
bowl. Turn to coat. Season using
garlic powder, pepper, salt, along
with Parmesan.

d. Place fries in a single line on a baking sheet lined with parchment paper. Bake 30–35 minutes, stirring midway, till golden brown.

e. Sprinkle fresh parsley on top and serve hot.

Nutritional Info

Amount per serving

About 1½ cups serving size
Calories

163; total fat: 5g; saturated fat: 1.1g; protein: 4g; carbohydrates:

25g fiber

2.7g sugar

1g added sugar

Zero grams sodium 191 mg

iii. Vegan Potato-Leek Soup

The health benefits of this soup aren't limited to vegans. According to studies, eating more plant-based foods including this dish may lower blood pressure, heart disease, and cancer risk. In fact, a recent study indicated that a plant-based diet reduced prostate cancer risk by 19% and mortality by 47% in males under 65.

Ingredients or components:

-Use 3 tablespoons of extra-virgin olive oil.

-4 leeks, white as well as light green sections only, roughly sliced 1 rib celery, cut into pieces 3 cloves, garlic, chopped 2 lbs Yukon gold potatoes, and skin on, ½-inch chunks

-4 cups low-sodium veggie broth

-1 tsp dry thyme

-One teaspoon of dried rosemary

-½ teaspoon ground coriander seeds, 2 bay leaves, 1 cup unscented soy milk

-2-tsp kosher salt

-½ tsp freshly crushed black pepper

Directions:

a. Add oil, leeks, celery, as well as garlic to a big stockpot over medium heat. Stir constantly until vegetables are tender, approximately 10 minutes.

b. Simmer potatoes, broth, coriander, rosemary, thyme, plus bay leaves. Cover, reduce heat, and simmer 20 minutes till potatoes are very soft.

c. Stop cooking. After cooling, drain bay leaves and purée soup employing an immersion or tabletop blender.

d. Add soy milk to stockpot and simmer over medium heat. Add salt and pepper as well as serve.

Nutritional Info

Amount per serving

Size of serving1 cup: 173 calories, 173 fat.

Six grams of saturated fat, 0.8 grams of protein, and four grams of carbs.

29g fiber, 3.3g sugar, 4g added sugar, 0g sodium, 400mg

iv. Herb Potato Salad

According to the USDA, potato salad commonly incorporates mayo, which is heavy in calories, salt, and saturated fat. Instead, this version uses olive oil, which has monounsaturated fatty acids that may lessen heart disease risk, study shows. A study found that cooking and cooling potatoes makes certain starch resistant. Another study found that resistant starch is hard to digest as well as has less calories and carbs.

Ingredients

-2 lb baby potatoes, halved

-2 tablespoons extra-virgin olive oil

-A 1/4 of a cup of white-like wine vinegar

-1-tbsp Dijon mustard

-3/4 tsp kosher salt

-¼ tsp newly ground black pepper

-¼ cup chopped red onion

-3 tablespoons capers

-2 tbsp chopped fresh dill

-2 tbsp chopped fresh basil or just parsley

Directions:

a. Soak potatoes in a big stockpot of cold water. Boil on medium-high. Cover and boil until potatoes are fork-tender, 12–15 minutes. Drain and chill.

b. Mix oil, vinegar, mustard sauce, salt, as well as pepper in a small bowl. Toss potatoes gently to coat.

c. Add onion, capers, dill, as well as basil and serve.

Nutritional Info

Amount per serving

Serving size: 1⅓ cups. Calories: 156.

Total fat: Five grams of saturated fat, 0.6 grams of protein, and three grams of carbs.

Contains 29g fiber, 3g sugar, 0g added sugar, and 350mg sodium.

v. Veg-Packed Baked Potato

Dinner can be made quickly with baked potatoes. The microwave is the fastest way to "bake" potatoes. Baked potatoes are generally topped with dairy products, bacon, sour cream, as well as butter, but they can also support nutritious components. They're topped with a USDA-recommended spinach salad for fiber and iron.

Ingredients:

-4 medium potatoes with russet skins

-3 tablespoons olive oil, divided

-One pinch kosher salt

-1 pinch freshly crushed black pepper

-Two cups baby spinach ½ finely sliced yellow bell pepper

-1/4 cup crumbled feta

-2 tablespoons sliced sun-dried tomatoes

-1/4 cup walnut halves

-3-tablespoon balsamic vinegar

-1 finely sliced scallion for garnish

Directions:

a. Scrub and pierce potatoes thoroughly. Place potatoes upon a microwave-safe plate as well as microwave at high power for 6 minutes. Microwave potatoes for 6 additional minutes after flipping. When a knife easily enters the middle of every potato, they are prepared. If not, microwave for two minutes beginning at a time until potato center is cooked.

b. Keep potato sides together when halving. Add a tablespoon of olive oil along with salt & pepper. Evenly distribute spinach, pepper pieces, feta, sun-dried tomatoes, along with walnut pieces among potatoes.

c. Apply remaining olive oil plus balsamic vinegar to each potato. Sprinkle scallions before serving.

Nutritional Info

Amount per serving

In a serving size of one potato, the calories are 351, the total fat is 17g, the saturated fat is 3.3g, and the protein is 8g.

44g fiber, 5.5g sugar, 5g added sugar, 0g sodium, 172mg

vi. Mashed Potatoes with Broccoli Pesto

Mash Yukon gold potatoes for a velvety texture without butter or milk. For a lump-free mash, cut the potatoes the same size as well as start them in cold water. One study says a broccoli recipe adds folate, vitamin C, plus vitamin K for minimal calories. Tasteful pesto uses olive oil or other unsaturated fats.

Ingredients

-Cut 2 pound Yukon gold potatoes into ½" chunks.

-One medium broccoli bunch, chopped very small

-2 minced garlic cloves, ¼ cup shredded Parmesan cheese

-1/4 cup basil pesto

-1-tsp kosher salt

-One-fourth teaspoon of newly ground black pepper, adding to taste

Directions:

a. Put potatoes in a big stockpot over a medium-high flame and cover with 2 inches of water. Cover the saucepan and boil.

b. After water boils, simmer potatoes for 10–12 minutes until tender but not done. Add broccoli, cover, and simmer for 4–5 minutes until brilliant green and tender. Reserve ½ cup of cooking water after draining.

c. Add saved water and the remaining components to drained veggies in stockpot. Use a potato mashing tool to blend the ingredients without overmixing.

Nutritional Info

Amount per serving

Serving size:

¾ cup Calories: 203

Total fat: 6g Saturated fat: 1.3g
Protein: 7g Carb

Contains 35g fiber, 5.6g sugar,
and 3g added sugar.

Zero grams Sodium: 416mg

vii. Potato Skin Bites Are Healthy

Potato peels are another great
potato dish. In contrast, this recipe
employs cheese as a condiment.
Mushrooms are rich in umami, the
fifth taste after sweet, sour, salty,

as well as bitter. According to a study, adding them to a recipe adds a delicious, meaty flavor without the health risks.

Ingredients

-1 pound fresh potatoes, ¾ cup minced baby portobello mushrooms

-2 chopped garlic cloves

-2 tablespoons extra-virgin olive oil

-1/2 tsp kosher salt

-Black pepper, for tasting

-One pinch chopped red pepper

-2 tablespoons freshly grated

-Parmesan cheese, along with more for garnish

-Optional fresh parsley garnish

Directions:

a. Pre-heat oven to 450°F.

Thoroughly scrub and fork-prick potatoes. Arrange on a microwave-safe pan and microwave for 5 minutes until a knife can easily enter the center. Cool potatoes until easily handled after cooking.

b. Slice every potato in half along with placing it on a baking sheet lined with parchment. Add mushrooms, garlic, and olive oil. Add pepper, salt, crushed red pepper, plus cheese.

c. Bake till cheese melts, 7–10 minutes. If using, put Parmesan and parsley on top and serve.

Nutritional Info

Per-serving calorie count

166 total fat

8g saturated fat

About 1.6g of protein

Contains 4g of carbs.

22 g fiber

2.6g sugar

1g added sugar

Zero grams Sodium: 231mg

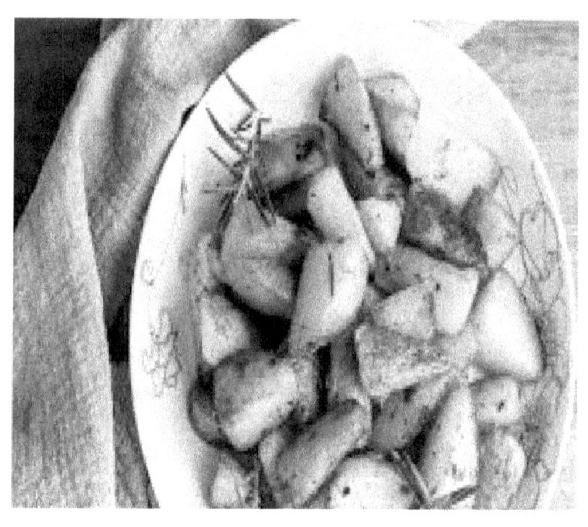

CHAPTER 5

AMAZING FACTS ABOUT POTATO DIET AND FAQS

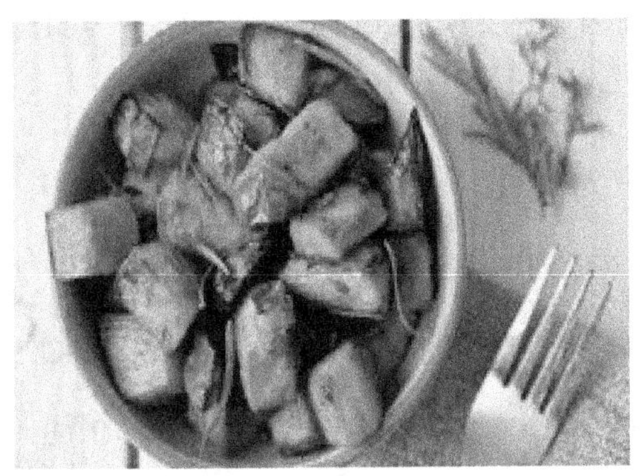

Can potatoes assist you lose weight?

Potatoes include resistant starch and fiber, keeping one full for longer period. They inhibit overeating.

You probably think of French fries, crispy potato chips, aloo tikki, and other deep-fried foods when you think of potatoes. No wonder we link potatoes with unhealthy stuff. Potatoes have a bad reputation as a fatty food because of this, and people trying to reduce weight and those with diabetes are advised to avoid them. Potatoes aren't bad if eaten properly.

Potatoes include elements that make them a good weight loss food.

Instead of being high in calories, potatoes can become unhealthy according to how they are cooked.

How potatoes prevent overeating

Potatoes include elements that make them a good weight loss food. Potatoes' fiber and resistant starch keep one satiated longer. Meaning it prevents overeating.

When you remain satiated, you really eat lesser caloric meal which is apparent on the weight size.

Potatoes increase metabolism

Potatoes include Potato Protease Inhibitors-2, which release Cholecystokinin to make you feel full.

NOTE: On top of that, potatoes also are high in antioxidants termed polyphenols, which boost the body's metabolism by burning down sugars at an increased rate,

How potatoes promote weight loss?

Abundant potassium in potatoes prevents water retention and aids weight loss.

Potatoes have been shown to shrink fat cells.

No one food will assist you gain or lose weight without a calorie restriction diet, and how we eat them is crucial.

Eating potatoes properly

Eating deep-fried potato snacks or fries clearly isn't the most beneficial way, but you are able to opt for methods including air-frying, baking, boiling, as well as roasting to have optimal benefits.

Alternatives to unhealthy potato snacks are always possible. Baked potato chips with olive oil can replace fried or deep-fried crisps.

You may make potato a great weight loss friend if you consume it appropriately.

Further Potato Frequently Asked Questions

Are potatoes good for athletes' diets?

Yes. A medium (that is, 5.3 ounces) skin-on potato has 620 mg of potassium, 26 grams of carbs and 110 calories for energy, crucial nutrients for athletes along with vigorous individuals.

Potatoes Healthy For You?

Yes. Potatoes are naturally cholesterol-free, fat-free, and low in sodium. Additionally, potatoes are rich in vitamin C and potassium when eaten with the skin. Foods high in potassium yet low in sodium, like potatoes, may lower the risk of elevated blood pressure as well as stroke.

Are All Potato Nutrients in The Skin?

No. Although the potato skin contains around half of the amount of dietary fiber, the vast majority of nutrients are located inside the potato itself.

Do the nutritional contents of the seven potato types differ?

There are about 200 potato types sold in the US. These potato cultivars fall into seven different groups: russet, white, red, yellow, blue/purple, fingerling, and tiny.

The dietary differences are minimal, but potatoes contain antioxidants such vitamin C, carotenoids, and anthocyanins.

Potato varieties determine quantity and types. Include a variety of potato kinds (e.g., reds, purples, yellows, russets) in your dietary regimen.

What is the distinction between sweet and white potatoes?

Both sweet potato and white potatoes include essential nutrients like protein (2 g vs. 3 g), potassium, and vitamin B6, contributing to a balanced, nutrient-dense diet.

Both have similar calorie, fiber, protein, and vitamin B6 levels. The potassium content of white potatoes is higher (620 mg vs. 440 mg), but sweet potatoes are rich in the nutrient such as vitamin A (that is, 120% of the recommended intake). Both are rich in vitamin C, with white potatoes providing 45%

of the recommended intake and sweet potatoes 30%.

Are Potatoes Rich In Carbs?

Yes. Potatoes are carb-heavy. A medium 5.3-ounce potato with skin has 26 g of carbohydrate.

Potatoes Fattening?

5.3-ounces skin-on potato provides 110 calories plus no fat.

According to studies, gaining weight occurs when individuals consume more energy than they burn.

How Long Does A Potato Cook?

Potatoes have hundreds of varieties. Preparation time varies per recipe and potato type, from minutes to an hour. For an instant stovetop supper, try smaller types and use the oven to speed up potato cooking.

How to Store Potatoes?

-Keep potatoes within a cool, ventilated area.

-Refrigerated temperatures below 50°F convert potato starch to sugar, causing a sweet taste and coloring when cooked. Allowing potatoes to reheat to room temp before cooking can reduce discolouration if refrigerated.

-Keep away from hot locations (under the sink or near major appliances) and exposed to sunlight (regarding the countertop).

-Perforated plastic and paper bags provide optimal shelf life.

-Do not expose potatoes to light.

-Don't wash potatoes or produce before storing.

-Dampness accelerates rotting.

How are potatoes grown?

The US potato crop is grown in practically all states, with half coming from Idaho, North Dakota, Washington, Wisconsin, Minnesota, Oregon, Maine, California, Colorado, as well as Michigan.

Potatoes are harvested mostly in September and October.

CHAPTER 6

IS POTATO REGIMEN GOOD HEALTH WISE? AND CONCLUSION

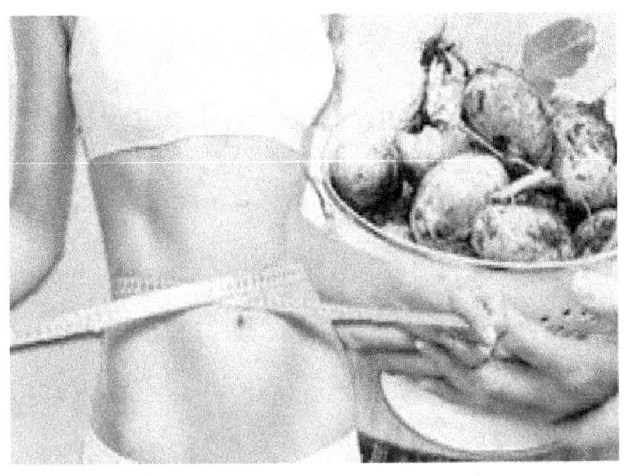

Is the Potato Cuisine Healthy?

Potatoes do not meet the 2020-2025 USDA Dietary Guidelines for Americans. The guidelines recommend eating potatoes as a starchy vegetable, but they also recommend eating from the key food groups. Potato eaters skip five out of six food groups.

The potato meal is high-fiber. The USDA recommends 28–34 grams of fiber daily for adults.

The potato regimen is minimal in sodium and fat. While salt is acceptable on the potato nutrition, it is discouraged. The potato regimen is low in sodium because potatoes are extremely low in sodium plus users can add minimal or no salt for taste. Though much sodium can harm health, it is important for fluid equilibrium, muscle, and nerve function.

Misconception: you must cut the amount of calories you consume every day to 1,200 to lose weight. This is far below the USDA's 1,600–2,000-calorie daily recommed for women and 2,000–2,400 for males.

Potato diet calories are not set. Eating until full is encouraged, thus followers may eat greater or lesser than recommended.

Mono diets like the potato diet may cause short-term weight loss but are unsustainable and may cause nutritional deficits.

CONCLUSION

Potatoes are a popular source of resilient starch, minerals, vitamins, and fiber. Yet, too much of something can be detrimental. A balanced diet includes nutrient-rich and enjoyable foods. On the potato diet, moderation is not allowed. However, devotees eat potatoes in big numbers.

Remember that many diets don't work, especially long-term, and you may not need one. I don't support fad diets or unrealistic weight loss approaches, but I provide the facts so you may make an informed decision based on your dietary requirements, genetic blueprint, budget, as well as goals.

Understand that losing weight isn't the same as achieving your fittest self, and that there are various ways to achieve health. Fitness, sleep, and other aspects of life also affect health. The optimum diet is balanced and lifestyle-friendly.

THE END.